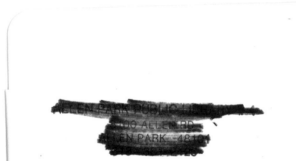
616.92 R
TWEEN

MAXINE ROSALER

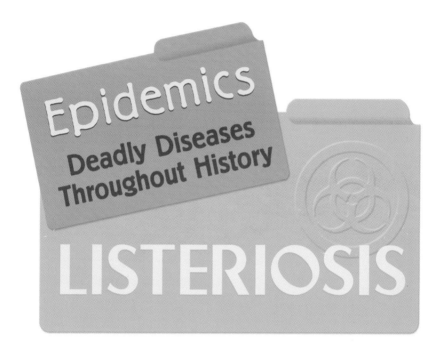

Epidemics
Deadly Diseases
Throughout History

LISTERIOSIS

The Rosen Publishing Group, Inc.
New York

Published in 2004 by The Rosen Publishing Group, Inc.
29 East 21st Street, New York NY 10010

First Edition

Library of Congress Cataloging-in-Publication Data

Rosaler, Maxine.
Listeriosis / by Maxine Rosaler.
    p. cm. — (Epidemics)
Summary: Discusses the symptoms, effects, outbreaks, and prevention of listeriosis, a disease caused by eating contaminated
food, and examines how scientists track its source.
Includes bibliographical references and index.
ISBN 0-8239-4202-3 (library bdg.)
1. Listeriosis—Juvenile literature. [1. Listeriosis. 2. Diseases.
3. Epidemics.] I. Title. II. Series.
RC155 .R67 2003
616.9′2—dc21

2002153250

Manufactured in the United States of America

Cover image: A colorized micrograph of *Listeria*

CONTENTS

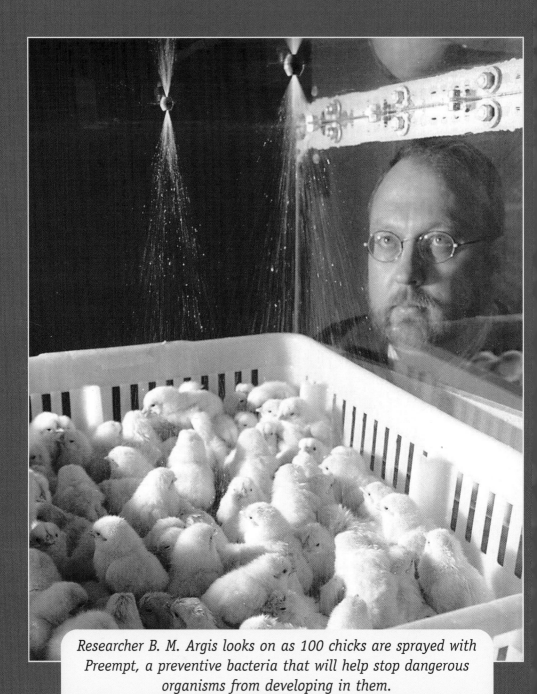

Researcher B. M. Argis looks on as 100 chicks are sprayed with *Preempt, a preventive bacteria that will help stop dangerous organisms from developing in them.*

INTRODUCTION

The sanitation conditions at Sara Lee's Bil Mar meat processing plant were not good. There were scraps of old meat lodged in equipment that plant managers had said were clean and ready for production. There were turkey carcasses smudged with feces waiting to be processed into lunch meats and hot dogs. Rust, plastic chips, meat shavings, and other debris could be found in food along the processing lines. Hanging above the assembly line of hot dogs were pipes on which beads of water would form and collect. Occasionally a droplet would fall onto the hot dogs just before they were about to be packaged and shipped out to grocery stores, where unsuspecting customers would purchase them and bring them home to serve to their families.

The United States Department of Agriculture (USDA), which is responsible for monitoring meat processing plants to make sure they are safe, had charged Bil Mar with many violations in the past. During the first six months of 1998 alone, the USDA had cited the plant for 112 violations. The problem with the pipes was of special concern to the USDA. The droplets falling onto the hot dogs could be teeming with dangerous disease-causing bacteria. Moist environments are ideal conditions for some bacteria to thrive and multiply. The conditions at Bil Mar were so bad that the USDA shut it down in November 1997. The Department of Agriculture rarely goes so far as to shut a plant down, but Bil Mar had too many dangerous violations for the USDA to allow it to continue producing food.

Anxious to get back to business, Bil Mar hurried to make enough improvements for the USDA to allow it to reopen that same month, but, as it soon became apparent, not many improvements were made. The problems with sanitation had by no means been taken care of. Many of the same problems persisted, including ones with the refrigeration unit. Ultimately, the sanitation unit was replaced.

However, as it turned out, the removal of the air-conditioning unit had actually resulted in making conditions at the plant much worse. Tests done after the unit was removed showed a sharp increase in the presence of bacteria. Four months later, a mysterious epidemic swept the country. The outbreak encompassed twenty-two states. Eighty people became seriously ill, and there were fifteen deaths, as well as six stillbirths or miscarriages. The source of the outbreak was eventually traced back to the Bil Mar plant. Though the exact cause of the outbreak was never proved, the removal of the air-conditioning unit was eventually blamed. Scientists said the removal of the unit had stirred up a lot of dust, which is known to be a good hiding place for bacteria.

The epidemic turned out to be listeriosis, which results from exposure to the bacterium *Listeria*, one of the deadliest food-borne bacteria known to exist.

1

LISTERIOSIS: A SHORT HISTORY

No one can say exactly when people first realized that food could make them sick, but researchers believe that people figured it out very early. Dating as far back as prehistoric times, evidence has been found indicating that people took measures to prevent food from spoiling. The Roman philosopher Lucretius, from the first century BC, went so far as to suggest that disease might be caused by invisible living creatures. At the time, few people accepted his theory.

At the beginning of the nineteenth century, many people believed that when food spoiled it produced chemical poisons that could cause illness. They called these poisons "ptomaines," from the Greek word *ptoma*, meaning "corpse."

However, what all our ancestors were referring to was in fact bacteria, those tiny invisible creatures that were not discovered until the late 1800s by two men, Louis Pasteur and Robert Koch. The discovery of bacteria marked the beginning of people's understanding of how spoiled food could cause illness.

The first bacterium that was found to cause illness was discovered by a German scientist named A. Gartner in 1888. He was studying an outbreak of meat poisoning that occurred in Frankenhausen, Germany, which killed one man and caused fifty-one illnesses. Gartner analyzed the infected meat and discovered a new type of bacterium, which he named *Bacillus enteritidis*. The bacterium was later renamed *Salmonella enteritidis*, or *Salmonella* for short.

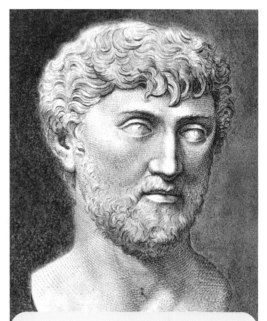

Roman poet and philosopher Lucretius theorized in the first century BC that organisms invisible to the naked eye might cause disease.

Another important discovery was made soon afterward in 1895 when Emile van Ermengem, a professor at the University of Ghent in Belgium, discovered the bacterium that causes the disease known as botulism. He named the bacterium *Bacillus botulinus* (now called *Clostridium botulinum*). Van Ermengem showed that this bacterium could grow and multiply in oxygen-free containers and that botulism itself is actually caused by a powerful poison, or toxin, produced by the microbe.

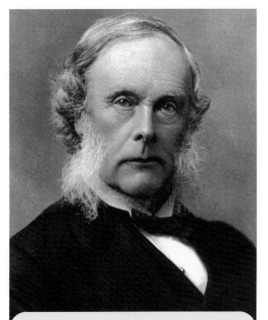

Dr. Joseph Lister was a medical pioneer who discovered the importance of sterilizing surgical instruments.

The Discovery Of *Listeria*

In the 1920s, an epidemic broke out among guinea pigs and rabbits that puzzled veterinarians. Scientists got to work, and in 1926, a team of scientists headed by Dr. Everitt Murray discovered the bacterium. They called it *Bacterium monocytogenes*. It was later renamed *Listeria monocytogenes* in honor of Dr. Joseph Lister, the doctor who discovered the need for surgeons to sterilize their instruments before operations in order

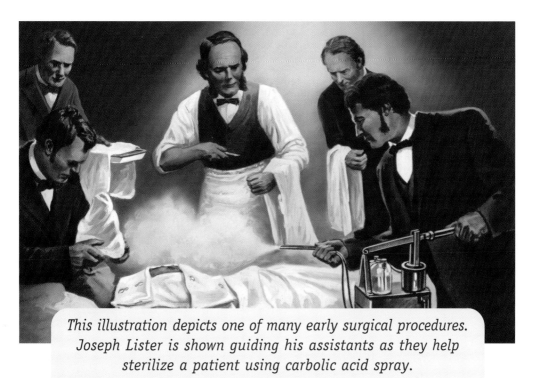

This illustration depicts one of many early surgical procedures. Joseph Lister is shown guiding his assistants as they help sterilize a patient using carbolic acid spray.

to prevent infection. The disease that *Listeria* causes was named listeriosis.

Ideas about listeriosis have gone through many changes over the years. When it was first discovered, scientists believed that it was only a disease of animals because there were no known human cases. But this changed in 1929 when the first human case of listeriosis was detected.

Throughout the 1930s, there was a dramatic increase in human cases of listeriosis. The increase in human cases happened at the same time as an increase in animal cases, which led scientists to believe that animals were spreading the disease to humans. Another reason for scientists to believe that animals were spreading the disease to humans was the fact that it was mostly farm workers who seemed to be coming down with the disease.

Scientists had to change their minds about listeriosis yet again when people who lived in the city, who had no contact with infected animals, started coming down with the disease. It began to dawn on public health officials that farm animals weren't the only carriers of listeriosis. But it wasn't until decades later, during the 1980s, when scientists figured out that people could get listeriosis by eating food that was contaminated with *Listeria*.

The Food Supply

A series of outbreaks that occurred during the 1980s forced scientists and government officials to finally admit that listeriosis was a serious problem that had to be tracked down immediately.

First, in 1981, there was an outbreak in Nova Scotia, Canada, that resulted in 41 cases including 18 deaths. Most of the victims who died were infants. Then, in 1983, an outbreak occurred in Boston, which resulted in 49 cases, including 14 deaths. In 1985, there was an outbreak in Los Angeles that resulted in 142 cases, including 48 deaths, 10 of whom were newborns.

All these outbreaks were traced back to infected food. The 1981 outbreak was traced to *Listeria* found on coleslaw that had been made from cabbage grown in fields fertilized with manure from *Listeria*-infected sheep. The 1983 outbreak was traced to milk that had not been adequately pasteurized. But it was not until the 1985 outbreak, the most deadly of the bunch, that researchers were finally convinced that the outbreak was the result of food-borne listeriosis. The 1985 outbreak was eventually traced back to equipment at the now-defunct Jalisco Mexican Products, which had manufactured contaminated cheese that people had consumed.

Federal investigators discovered that the equipment at the plant was contaminated with *Listeria* even after it had been cleaned and sanitized. In addition, they found that the milk that had been used to manufacture the cheese had not been adequately pasteurized. Pasteurization, a process that uses very high heat to kill germs, is known to be effective in killing *Listeria*. After 1985, the USDA and the Food and Drug Administration (FDA), which is responsible for ensuring the safety of food and drugs in the United States, began testing dairy products for *Listeria*.

The 1985 outbreak was the first that involved cheese, and for a while it was thought that only plants that processed dairy products were vulnerable to infection with *Listeria*. But in 1989, the Centers for Disease Control and Prevention (CDC), which is responsible for monitoring diseases in the United States and heading all investigations into outbreaks, traced a case of listeriosis to turkey hot dogs. The USDA started testing processed, ready-to-eat meats for the bacteria. The testing was eventually expanded to include seafood and meat salads and spreads.

Shortly after the 1980s outbreaks, the CDC classified listeriosis as a "reportable disease," one of the ten diseases for which state public health departments are obligated to notify the CDC because of their level of seriousness.

LEARNING FROM LISTERIOSIS OUTBREAKS

Cases of listeriosis are usually isolated incidents and not epidemics. When illnesses occur separately like this, they are called "sporadic." Sporadic cases of listeriosis don't leave as many clues as large outbreaks, so their sources often remain mysterious.

Large outbreaks of listeriosis are easier to investigate since they allow researchers to collect a lot of information that might lead to discovering the source. Even with large outbreaks, though, investigators may be unable to figure out what went wrong.

An outbreak in Switzerland between 1983 and 1987, for example, involved at least 123 cases, including 34 deaths (there were 16 cases in 1983, 24 in 1984, 13 in 1985, 28 in 1986, and 42 in 1987). The outbreak was eventually traced to contamination of Vacherin Mont d'Or cheese, but it wasn't until more than a year after the outbreak that the cheese was discovered to be the source.

In 1992, an outbreak of listeriosis in France resulted in 279 illnesses, leading to 22 miscarriages and 63 deaths. It was attributed to the consumption of pork tongue in aspic (a jelly produced by the juices of fish or meat bones).

Poorly pasteurized chocolate milk was the cause of a 1995 outbreak in Illinois that sickened 45 of the 60 people who had consumed the milk. There were no deaths reported. The particular strain of *Listeria* that had caused the sickness was finally tracked down to a drain at the manufacturing plant and to unopened packs of the implicated milk. The inadequate pasteurization of the milk was blamed on defective equipment. Milk was pasteurized and then moved to a holding tank before individual containers were filled. Defects in the holding tank prevented the milk from being refrigerated.

An outbreak of listeriosis in France in 1995 affected 17 people, including 9 pregnant women. The infection resulted in two stillbirths and two miscarriages, and one elderly person was reported to have fallen into a coma as a result. Brie de Meaux soft cheese was reported to be the cause of the outbreak.

(Continued on page 16)

15

In 1998, there was an outbreak of listeriosis in the United States that included 22 states and resulted in 101 cases of listeriosis, 15 of whom died. There were also 6 miscarriages or stillbirths. The cause of the outbreak was traced to hot dogs and deli meats produced by a Sara Lee processing plant. Construction dust that was infected with *Listeria* was believed to have contaminated the product in the packing room. As a result of the outbreak, the plant recalled 35 million pounds of hot dogs, including Ball Park Franks and lunch meat, because of contamination with *Listeria*.

Sara Lee pleaded guilty to a federal misdemeanor charge of selling adulterated meat. The company paid a $200,000 fine and promised to spend $3 million on food safety research. The recall cost the company $76 million. In addition, victims sought millions of dollars in damages. So far, Sara Lee has settled these lawsuits for approximately $5 million.

An outbreak of listeriosis in 2002 killed 7 people and sickened dozens of others in 7 states in the northeastern United States. The outbreak was traced to a meat processing plant belonging to Pilgrim's Pride, the second largest poultry producer in the United States, although the exact cause of the contamination is not yet known. This outbreak resulted in the biggest recall of meat in the history of the U.S. Department of Agriculture. More than 27 million pounds of meat were taken out of supermarket refrigerators and warehouses, and customers were asked to return the meat to the stores where they had purchased it.

2

THE SPREAD OF LISTERIOSIS

Pathogens are microorganisms that cause disease, and *Listeria* is one of the deadliest. In 1999 the CDC reported that of all the food-borne pathogens tracked by the CDC, *Listeria* had the second highest death rate, about 20 percent.

Listeria is found everywhere in nature—in soil, decaying vegetation, sewage, dust and water. Since it is so widely present in the environment, it is impossible to prevent animals from coming in contact with the bacterium, contracting it, and eventually spreading it.

How Listeriosis Is Contracted

People get listeriosis by simply eating food contaminated with *Listeria*. Babies can also be born

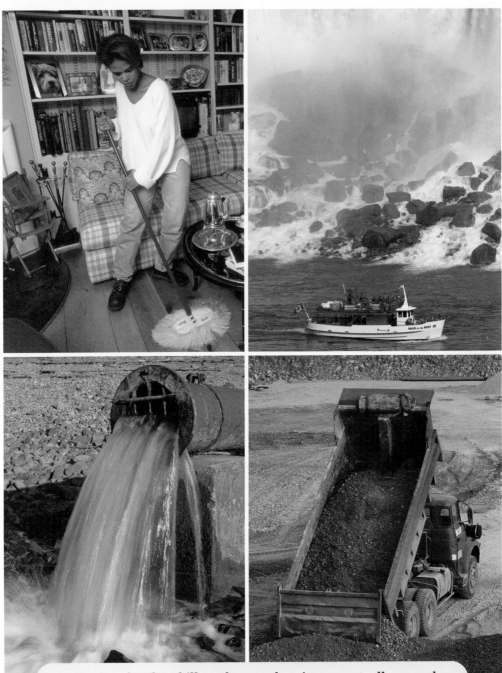

Listeria *is a hard-to-kill pathogen that is present all around us, whether in the home, in the water, in natural settings, or in man-made environments.*

with listeriosis if their mothers eat contaminated food during pregnancy. Though white blood cells (one of the body's protections against infection) will kill *Listeria*, they are defenseless against listeriosis. In fact, *Listeria* will use the white blood cells against the body. First it will invade the white blood cells and kill them. Then, once inside, *Listeria* will use these cells as vehicles for traveling through the bloodstream to spread the infection throughout the body.

Symptoms

The symptoms of listeriosis vary from individual to individual and depend on how susceptible a person is to the disease. Healthy people may experience symptoms such as fever, chills, fatigue, nausea, vomiting, and diarrhea. And the symptoms might go no further than that. Infected pregnant women may experience only a mild, flu-like illness, even when the illness results in miscarriage or the death of their babies.

If infection spreads to the nervous system, which, for reasons unknown, is very susceptible to the disease, symptoms such as headache, stiff neck, confusion, loss of balance, or convulsions may occur. Also, when the bacteria invade the central nervous system, a brain infection called meningitis can occur. Septicemia (bacteria in the bloodstream, or blood poisoning) is the other more serious result of listeriosis.

It can take anywhere from one to six weeks for a person who has eaten contaminated food to develop listeriosis, though flu-like symptoms may occur twelve hours after eating *Listeria*-contaminated food. The amount of *Listeria* that is needed to infect a person with listeriosis is unknown.

Listeriosis can be diagnosed by testing the victim's blood and spinal fluid, and it can be treated with antibiotic drugs such as penicillin or ampicillin.

A Very Tough Bug

According to the Mayo Clinic, *Listeria* is the toughest food-borne bacterium to kill. It can survive in environments that would kill most other bacteria. It can resist heat, salt, and the kinds of acids that are commonly used in food preservatives better than most other organisms, and it can grow in temperatures as low as 1°F to as high as 113°F. Only temperatures above 160°F and below 0°F can kill the bacteria.

Refrigeration has always been one of the food industry's standard safety defenses, but it is useless against *Listeria*. While refrigeration stops most bacteria from growing, *Listeria* thrives in cold environments. It is what is known as psychrophilic, or

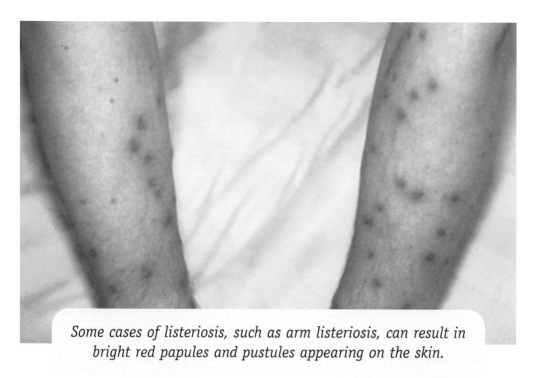

Some cases of listeriosis, such as arm listeriosis, can result in bright red papules and pustules appearing on the skin.

cold-loving. While bacteria stop growing when temperatures fall below 0°F, other food-borne bacteria stop growing when temperatures fall below 40°F.

Dangerous Foods

Listeria has been detected in a variety of foods. Vegetables can become contaminated with *Listeria* by being fertilized with manure from infected animals. Since an animal can often have listeriosis without showing any symptoms, the meat and dairy products that they produce can be infected with *Listeria* without anyone realizing it.

High temperatures usually kill *Listeria*. But processed foods such as cold cuts, which are usually not heated, are particularly vulnerable to being infected with the bacteria. Unpasteurized milk or foods made from unpasteurized milk are also prime targets.

People at Risk

Though listeriosis is not a serious disease for healthy people, it is very serious for people with weakened immune systems or diseases such as cancer or diabetes, which often require them to take drugs that suppress their immune systems. People with AIDS are the most vulnerable; they are almost three hundred times more likely to get listeriosis than people with healthy immune systems.

Pregnant women are also especially vulnerable to listeriosis since *Listeria* has the ability to penetrate the usually impenetrable placenta. The infection passes directly from the mother's blood to the fetus. About one third of listeriosis cases happen during pregnancy.

3

OUTBREAKS

When it comes to tracing the source of a food-borne epidemic, researchers rely on the same kinds of skills and technology that police do when tracking down someone who has committed a violent crime. For example, each bacterium contains its own distinctive DNA, as all living things do. Just as DNA testing is used to track down the perpetrator of a crime, it is sometimes used to track down the particular strain, or type, of bacterium that is causing an outbreak.

Similarly, just as detectives collect clues by interviewing the victims and witnesses of a crime, investigators of a food epidemic interview the victims of the outbreaks, or people who were close to the victims, to discover what food the victims ate before they got sick, where they ate it, and where that food came from.

Discovering the Problem

In mid-October 1998, reports of listeriosis started appearing on the desk of Dr. Paul Mead, an epidemiologist at the CDC who oversaw investigations of food-borne illnesses. The first four came in from Tennessee, then five from Ohio, nine from New York, and one from Connecticut.

Each bacterium carries its own distinctive genetic fingerprint, or unique DNA structure. So the states that reported the listeriosis cases all sent in samples for genetic fingerprinting. The results of the tests showed that many of the listeriosis cases shared an extremely rare genetic fingerprint, which the researchers called the "E" strain. This meant that many of the victims had been attacked by the same strain of *Listeria*, which was a strong indication that many of the victims had eaten food that had come from a common source.

Convinced that an outbreak of listeriosis was indeed in the works, Dr. Mead got to work right away on launching an investigation into the cause of the outbreak. He sent out a nationwide alert via fax to state public health departments, telling them that there had been a sharp increase in the number of cases of listeriosis being reported. The faxes all told the state departments to be on the lookout for illnesses caused by *Listeria*.

The Hot Dog Connection

By December, the outbreak had spread to Massachusetts, Michigan, West Virginia, and Oregon. By this time, Dr. Mead had come up with another important finding: Many of the victims with the type E strain of listeriosis had remembered eating hot dogs.

There had been several cases of listeriosis reported in Ohio, and thinking that there might be some leads to be found there, Dr. Mead sent Dr. Eileen Dunne out to investigate. Dr. Dunne is an epidemic intelligence worker. Her job is to search for clues to find out what the cause of a particular epidemic might be, much like a detective.

The first thing Dr. Dunne did when she arrived in Ohio was to visit a nursing complex, located in a Cleveland suburb, where three cases of listeriosis had been reported. But after she discovered that the genetic fingerprints on the samples that had been taken from the nursing complex's residents did not match the fingerprint of the outbreak strain, she began to search elsewhere for clues. With the help of health workers at the local health department, she went door to door, interviewing people who had been diagnosed with listeriosis in the state.

One of the homes that Dr. Dunne visited was that of a woman who had recently given birth. The baby had

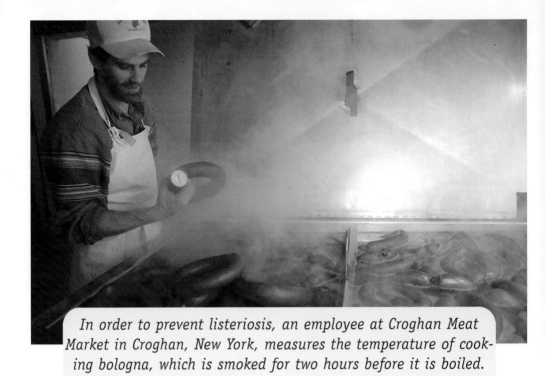

In order to prevent listeriosis, an employee at Croghan Meat Market in Croghan, New York, measures the temperature of cooking bologna, which is smoked for two hours before it is boiled.

been born prematurely, as a result of the mother having contracted listeriosis during her pregnancy. In the course of questioning the woman about what she remembered eating during the weeks before she gave birth, Dr. Dunne found out that the woman had eaten hot dogs. As luck would have it, it turned out the woman still had an open package of the hot dogs in her refrigerator. Dr. Dunne knew that this would be an important clue, and she quickly packed the hot dogs in ice and shipped them off to the CDC for testing.

In the meantime, health officials in states across the country had been spending weeks doing what Dr. Dunne had been doing: knocking on doors and asking people about what they remembered eating before they fell sick. Many of the people who had been interviewed also reported that they had eaten hot dogs. Furthermore, many of the victims remembered that the hot dogs they had eaten had been manufactured by Sara Lee. Sara Lee was the same company that had manufactured the hot dogs that Dr. Dunne found in the refrigerator of the woman in Ohio.

To alert state health departments across the country, Dr. Mead sent out the following e-mail: "Dear Colleagues, The pieces of the multistate *Listeria* puzzle appear to be falling into place . . . Hot dogs have a long shelf life (decades in my freezer), and we have good reason to believe that cases are ongoing . . . it is not clear that the company will feel that the data is strong enough to support a recall at this time. WE DESPERATELY NEED ADDITIONAL PRODUCT INFORMATION: brand names, establishment numbers, dates of production for both hot dogs and deli meats. We ask you to please redouble your efforts to get this information."

Seeking Out the Culprits

Sara Lee is a huge company, with several meat plants producing hot dogs under many different brand names scattered throughout the country. But the package of hot dogs that had been recovered from the young

According to federal investigators, managers of the Sara Lee processing plant that was found to be the source of the 1998 multistate outbreak of listeriosis knew that the plant had a problem with *Listeria* eight months before the outbreak occurred. Federal investigators also stated that not only were plant managers aware of the fact that the *Listeria* danger existed, they had tried to cover it up as well.

Employees told the federal investigators that they were warned to keep secret the fact that *Listeria* had been detected in the plant. According to statements that employees gave to federal investigators, plant managers told employees that "loose [lips] sink ships."

Evidence of listeriosis at the plant had been detected as early as six months before the outbreak occurred. Federal investigators found out that in addition to keeping the *Listeria* problem a secret, managers of the Bil Mar plant had a practice of trying to "skirt the law" by not testing the meat for *Listeria*. By not testing the meat, managers felt that they could always claim that they weren't responsible for shipping contaminated meat, since without testing, they couldn't know whether or not the meat was tainted with *Listeria*.

Federal investigators also reported that one former Bil Mar employee said that plant managers specifically directed laboratory technicians not to test for *Listeria*. The lab technicians were instead told to test only for conditions that might promote the growth of *Listeria*. Workers were also told to hide the lab test results in a special file that was to be withheld from the USDA.

mother's refrigerator contained an important clue that would allow CDC investigators to find out where the hot dogs originated: a manufacturer's code. This code led the CDC to Bil Mar Foods in Michigan.

But the CDC could still not be certain that Bil Mar was the source of the listeriosis outbreak. Even if the hot dogs did test positive for *Listeria*, this would still not be sufficient proof—the hot dogs could have been infected from other bacteria that lived in the woman's refrigerator.

Before accusing Bil Mar of being the source of the epidemic, the CDC investigators would have to conduct tests on the plant itself. Dr. Mead sent Dr. Dunne to Bil Mar to investigate. When she

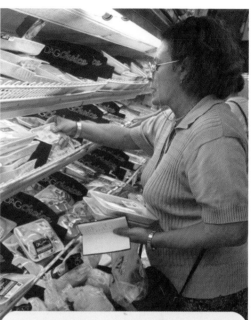

Manufacturers' codes allow the CDC and other agencies to track the movements of food products.

arrived at the plant, Dr. Dunne asked the plant managers if anything unusual had taken place during the previous six months. She inquired about plumbing problems, construction work, or other interruptions in

State health departments maintain lists of food-borne diseases that doctors, clinical laboratories, and hospitals are required by law to report to their local health departments. Since certain diseases, like listeriosis, take a long time to diagnose, doctors are cautioned against waiting until they know for sure that the patient has listeriosis before reporting the symptoms. Instead, they are urged to contact their health departments immediately when they suspect that a patient might have the disease. The earlier food-borne and other epidemic diseases are reported, the sooner the health departments can get to work on determining whether an outbreak is occurring. In addition, the sooner they begin, the sooner they can trace the source of the outbreak and save more people from contracting the disease.

After a local health department receives a report about an illness that is on the state health department's list of reportable illnesses, it is, in turn, required to report the case to the state health department. It is then up to the state health department to determine whether the illness needs further investigation.

If the state health department suspects that the illness is food-borne, it reports it to the CDC. If the CDC believes a food-borne outbreak might be in the works, it launches an investigation into the causes of the outbreak.

Still, despite the importance of reporting food-borne illnesses, doctors and labs often fail to report them to health departments. Since listeriosis is a rare disease, many doctors are not even aware of what it is, much less that they are required to report it. In addition, many

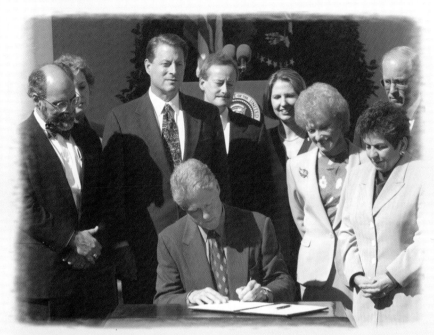

President Bill Clinton signs an initiative on October 2, 1997, that aims to improve the safety of imported and domestic agricultural products.

symptoms of listeriosis—diarrhea, fever, fatigue—are similar to those of many other diseases and conditions, and are therefore difficult to accurately diagnose.

"Far too many medical professionals are very uneducated when it comes to food-borne illness and what to look for, what to test for," says Nancy Donley, president of Safe Tables Our Priority (STOP), a national advocacy group for victims of food-borne illnesses.

the regular routine. Like a detective, she inquired about anything that might give her clues about the outbreak. As a result, Dr. Dunne uncovered one important fact: Construction workers had removed a defective refrigeration unit from the plant over the previous Fourth of July weekend. Furthermore, Dr. Dunne discovered that the refrigeration unit was located in the area of the plant where hot dogs were produced.

Plant managers explained to CDC investigators that the workers were unable to remove the unit in one piece. Instead, they had to saw it into individual pieces, which they dragged through the plant corridors, including a main hallway right outside the hot dog production area. CDC investigators ultimately learned that tests showed there had been a sharp increase in *Listeria* immediately following the removal of the air conditioner.

The CDC suspected that it was the removal of the air-conditioning unit that was to blame. Dangerous bacteria could have possibly been living in the ceiling, and removing the unit released these bacteria. If so, the construction workers might have spread dust carrying the *Listeria* bacteria throughout the plant when they dragged out the pieces of the unit. It was thought that when the plant reopened, steam from passing hot dogs went up to the ceiling, condensed, and dripped back down with the dangerous bacteria onto the hot dogs.

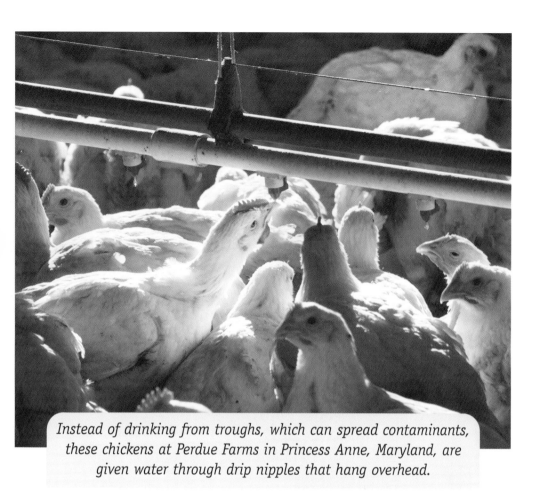

Instead of drinking from troughs, which can spread contaminants, these chickens at Perdue Farms in Princess Anne, Maryland, are given water through drip nipples that hang overhead.

All the clues pointed to this theory. Ironically, the dismantling of the refrigeration unit, which had been intended to correct a problem, had very likely created a much larger one. And though investigators were never able to find exact evidence to prove their theory, they remain convinced that this was the cause of the outbreak.

November 1997

The Bil Mar Foods plant in Zeeland, Michigan, is shut down for several days by the USDA because of condensation dripping in meat-processing areas.

January– June 1998

The USDA cites Bil Mar Foods repeatedly for continued condensation troubles, including fluids dripping from pipes and ceilings directly onto cooked meats.

July 26–28 1998

USDA cites poor sanitation at Bil Mar, saying some areas "appeared to have been neglected for a significant period of time." Bil Mar pledges improvement.

July Fourth weekend, 1998

Workers with chain saws cut apart a refrigeration unit in the Bill Mar hot-dog plant. Afterward, tests reveal elevated levels of bacteria.

October 20, 1998

CDC receives notice from Tennessee of four listeriosis cases and begins investigation. More cases are reported from Ohio, New York, and Connecticut.

December 3, 1998

CDC statistical analysis of victims' food histories shows a strong link between listeriosis and eating hot dogs.

December 15, 1998

With four known victims dead, CDC informs USDA and Sara Lee of preliminary finding that Bil Mar is the source of outbreak. Bil Mar continues production but stops shipping.

November 20, 1998

Lab results show eighteen victims were attacked by single strain of *Listeria* from common food source.

December 14, 1998

The CDC identifies three Sara Lee brands—Ball Park, Bryan, and Kahn—as likely sources of outbreak.

December 18, 1998
Following news reports, Sara Lee meets with USDA officials, who do not recommend recall.

December 22, 1998
Sara Lee announces recall of all meat produced at Bil Mar since July 4.

January 20, 1999
With death toll at fourteen, Sara Lee takes out newspaper ads reminding consumers of the recall.

December 21, 1998
CDC recommends recall to Sara Lee, warning if company waits for further lab results "more illnesses and deaths will likely occur."

December 25, 1998
Lab tests of unopened package of Bil Mar hot dogs confirm outbreak strain.

January 28, 1999
USDA issues first press release, adding several brand names to list of tainted meats.

March 3, 1999
Bil Mar resumes deli meat production.

May 25, 1999
USDA warns that fifty million consumers with immunity problems should not eat hot dogs or deli meats unless they are fully recooked.

June 23, 2001
Sara Lee pleads guilty to producing and distributing tainted meat and agrees to pay $4.4 million to settle civil and criminal charges.

May 7, 2000
President Bill Clinton announces preventive measures for meat processing plants to reduce listeriosis outbreaks by half by 2005.

September 17, 2002
Reports confirm that a single strain of listeriosis killed seven people and sickened dozens of others in seven states in the northeastern United States.

4

THE CULPRITS

Since *Listeria* can be found virtually everywhere, it can contaminate food at every step along the way to people's tables—from the farm, where it is harvested; to manufacturing plants, where it is processed and packaged; to the market, where it is sold. While it is important to guard against contamination at every stage of production, improving sanitation at the processing plants where food is produced is the best way of preventing listeriosis outbreaks. Most outbreaks occur when food producers do not take the proper measures to ensure that the food is free of *Listeria*. And most contamination occurs after food is processed and before it is packaged, so food producers need to pay especially careful attention to this stage of the operation.

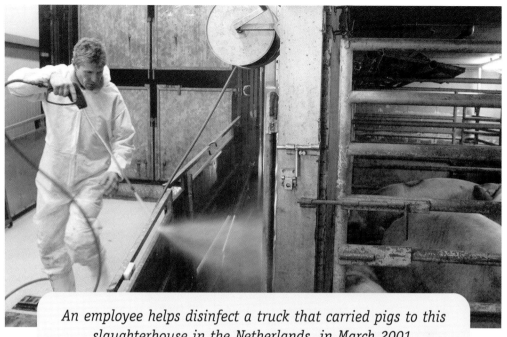

An employee helps disinfect a truck that carried pigs to this slaughterhouse in the Netherlands, in March 2001.

Hazard Analysis

Making sure that food producers run sanitary plants is on the top of the government's list for controlling *Listeria*. To this end, the USDA has created a safety system called the Hazard Analysis and Critical Control Point (HACCP) system, which all food producers are required to use.

The HACCP system provides plants with a guide for designing safety programs. Specifically, a HACCP program requires a plant to identify any problems, or potential problems, it may have with sanitation, and then to outline the steps for correcting them. With

Listeria, for example, where temperatures of 160°F are needed to kill the bacteria, a HACCP program would specify the cooking temperatures. Under HACCP, plants are also required to address issues such as plant layout and design, procedures for processing, and cleaning methods that are effective in killing *Listeria*.

HACCP, which went into effect in 1998, puts food safety into the hands of the plants themselves. Before it was created, government agencies had the primary responsibility for policing plant sanitation practices.

However, USDA meat inspectors say that the HACCP system turns over too much of the job of food safety to the companies. It also relies too much on the "honor system" for plants to guard against contamination. They complain that inspectors spend much more time looking over the plant's paperwork about its HACCP program than they do inspecting the plants themselves.

"We're not doing sanitation every day anymore," Rick Wolff, a USDA union official, said at a meeting of the USDA. "We're not doing a lot of things every day."

"You want to know where *Listeria* is coming from?" says Arthur Hughes, another USDA union official. "We are no longer monitoring sanitation. We're no longer doing these kinds of things. So, what happens as a result of that? *Listeria* is out of control." Because of

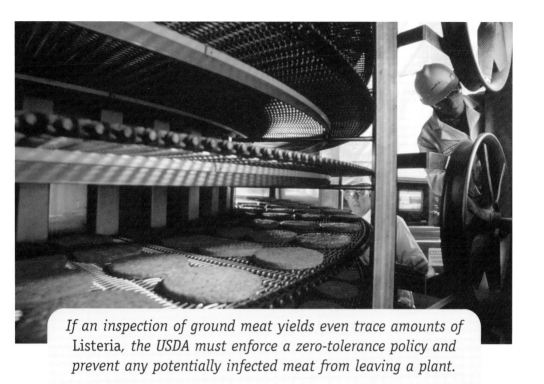

If an inspection of ground meat yields even trace amounts of Listeria, *the USDA must enforce a zero-tolerance policy and prevent any potentially infected meat from leaving a plant.*

this lack of guidelines regarding sanitation, some inspectors joke that HACCP stands for "Have a cup of coffee and pray."

A Zero-Tolerance Policy

Central to the USDA's efforts to control *Listeria* at food processing plants is what is known as the zero-tolerance policy. This means that when the federal inspectors who monitor processing plants find that a food product has been contaminated with any amount of *Listeria*—no matter how small—they do not allow the manufacturer of that food to ship the contaminated product out of the factory to the food markets. In 1987, in order to enforce its zero-tolerance policy, the USDA had its Food Safety and Inspection Service (FSIS) go into plants that it regulated to conduct random tests specifically for *Listeria*.

The government claims that the zero-tolerance policy is one of its most effective weapons against the spread of the disease, but not everyone agrees. Critics point out that testing for listeriosis is often done only once or twice a year. This, they say, is too infrequent for the zero-tolerance policy to have much effect.

Recall Policy

In addition to ordering the manufacturer not to send food to market if *Listeria* is found in it, the USDA can also ask the manufacturer of the contaminated product to do what is known as a voluntary recall—that is, the USDA will ask the company to tell the food markets to remove the contaminated products from store shelves and tell consumers to remove the products from their homes. The contaminated products would then be sent back to the manufacturer.

Before urging a company to do a recall, however, the USDA usually requires scientific evidence that contamination exists inside a plant—this means that areas of the plant have to test positive for *Listeria*, and the strains of *Listeria* at the plant would have to match the strains that were found in the victims, as well as the food that made them ill. The USDA Food Safety and Inspection Service has reported that the number-one cause of food recalls in 1999 was *Listeria*.

5

THE NEED FOR CHANGE

The 1998 outbreak of listeriosis shined a spotlight on the flaws in the nation's food safety system. After Bil Mar, the government committed itself to trying to fight *Listeria* more effectively and to find ways to prevent future outbreaks from occurring.

Before Bil Mar, USDA federal inspectors tested only thirty-five hundred samples of food products at meat processing plants each year. After Bil Mar, the USDA increased its testing of food for *Listeria* to five thousand per year. (According to some estimates, the USDA is now testing ten thousand samples per year.)

Before Bil Mar, packaged products were almost never tested for *Listeria*. After Bil Mar, the USDA started urging all processed meat producers to

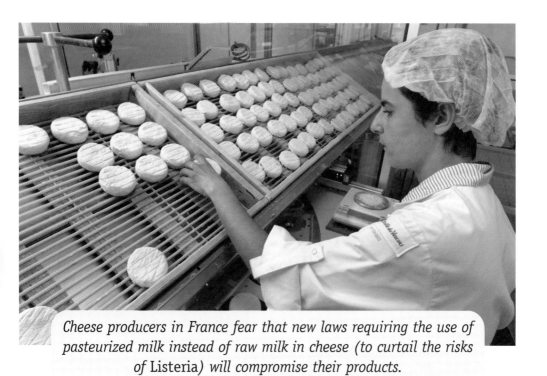

Cheese producers in France fear that new laws requiring the use of pasteurized milk instead of raw milk in cheese (to curtail the risks of Listeria*) will compromise their products.*

test work surfaces, equipment, and finished products specifically for listeria. The government also considered the *Listeria* threat to be so great that the USDA and the CDC issued warnings to people who were at risk of contracting the disease. The warnings advised these people to refrain from eating hot dogs or deli meats unless they recooked them until they were steaming hot. The agency also took steps to warn the at-risk groups against eating soft cheeses such as Brie, which are particularly vulnerable to *Listeria* contamination.

After the Bil Mar outbreak, the USDA directed plants to review their HACCP plans to make sure that they specifically addressed the problem of preventing *Listeria* in hot dogs and ready-to-eat meats, and federal inspectors reviewed those plans to see whether their plans for controlling *Listeria* were adequate.

While almost everyone agrees that these are all steps in the right direction, there are many consumer groups and government officials who feel that much more needs to be done to guard against this deadly bacterium.

Warning Labels

Consumer groups say that in addition to educating people about the dangers of eating certain foods, the USDA should require precooked foods such as hot dogs and lunch meats to carry warnings on their labels informing consumers that the products could contain dangerous, even deadly bacteria, and telling them about the need to cook these foods thoroughly before consumption. Critics say that it is misleading to label packaged deli and luncheon meats "cooked" and "ready-to-eat," since they could be deadly for at-risk groups if these people eat them without heating them.

A Call for More Testing

One of the most sweeping changes that is being sought is more testing. Critics say that every company that processes hot dogs and deli meats should be required to test its products and its processing plants for *Listeria*. Right now, if plants test for bacteria, they do so on a purely voluntary basis. Furthermore, critics say that the number of tests that the USDA does is too small to be effective. The USDA is responsible for overseeing the food safety at 6,200 meat plants. While some companies agree that food plants should be testing for *Listeria*, others are afraid of the idea. They worry that if a plant finds some of the bacteria in drains or on floors but not in foods, it might be pushed to do an unnecessary recall. In many cases, lawyers say that positive test results could be used against companies in court. Companies therefore will often choose not to test for *Listeria* at all, fearing what the consequences might be if they do detect the bacteria anywhere in the plant. This has led critics to dub the government's zero-tolerance policy a "don't look, don't find" policy.

Recalls

The government does not have the power to order a recall even when it finds out that a food product is contaminated with *Listeria*. Critics argue that if the government can order the recall of products such as unsafe cars, toys, and insecticides, it should have the power to order recalls of food that can kill people.

In the past, the USDA has been ineffective when asking for the authority to order food recalls. The food industry is opposed to mandatory recalls, and it has lobbied strongly against them. Some say that this is why efforts to give the USDA the power to order recalls have failed to date.

Senator Tom Harkin of Iowa, a Democrat who sits on the Agriculture Committee, wants the USDA to have more power over food safety. He has said that the government's lack of ability to enforce the laws that are designed to cover food safety "borders on the ridiculous."

Another long-standing problem with recalls has been the lack of publicity they are given. In the past, recalls were often conducted in secret in order to save the companies from negative publicity. For example, the USDA did not publicize the 1998 Sara Lee recall of thirty-five million pounds of hot dogs and lunch meats. Instead, they left it up to Sara Lee to tell people about the incident. In addition, Sara Lee greatly understated the nature of the recall. In a press release dated December 22, 1998, the company stated only that it was voluntarily recalling "specific production lots of hot dogs and other packaged meat products . . . The CDC has indicated it is studying whether some of these products might contain the *Listeria* bacteria."

The announcement made no mention of any illnesses or deaths, and it described the recall as a "precautionary measure." It did not describe the symptoms of listeriosis, except to say that it "affects primarily the elderly, pregnant women, newborns, and adults with weakened immune systems."

To address the problem with recalls, on February 1, 2000, the USDA passed a new federal food safety policy, which was designed to give the public more information about meat recalls. "An effective recall requires planning," says Philip Derfler, a deputy administrator at USDA's FSIS. "If they wait until they need to recall a product, it's too late."

The new policy urges companies to develop formal recall plans, to hold periodic recall drills, and to develop product coding systems that make it easier to track down products. Also, the policy states that in the event of a meat recall, federal regulators will issue a press release warning the public of the potential danger. The meat industry objects to this part of the policy, since they say it will unfairly subject companies to negative publicity.

Killing the Bug

Since *Listeria* contamination occurs most often between the time food has been processed and before it is packaged, food safety plans often focus on this stage of the production process.

One way of addressing this problem is to kill any lingering *Listeria* after meat is packaged. This can be done by treating products with radiation or heat after they have been sealed in packages.

In post-thermal processing, after it has been packaged, food is reheated to a temperature that is high enough to kill *Listeria* in the product. Similarly, food irradiation is the process of killing food-borne bacteria by exposing the food to levels of radiation. The radiation is strong enough to kill pathogens, but it is not strong enough to make the food radioactive. The radiant energy goes deeply into the food, killing microorganisms. It does so without raising the temperature of the food significantly.

The FDA requires that all irradiated foods be labeled with a symbol called the radura to inform consumers that the food they are buying has been irradiated. Adding chemicals to food that will kill or prevent the growth of *Listeria* is another method of fighting the bacterium. The chemicals used are natural salts and acids, such as sodium diacetate, sodium lactate, and potassium lactate. These food additives have been used as flavor enhancers for years.

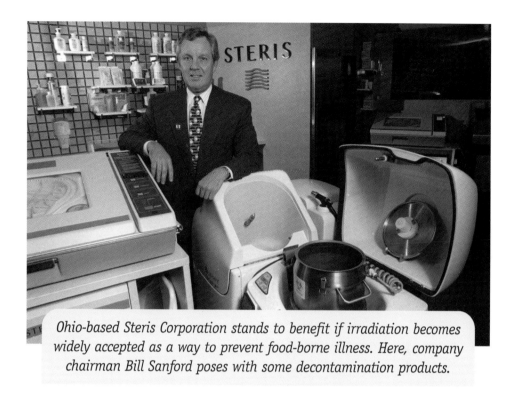

Ohio-based Steris Corporation stands to benefit if irradiation becomes widely accepted as a way to prevent food-borne illness. Here, company chairman Bill Sanford poses with some decontamination products.

A Growing Threat

The threat of contamination by *Listeria* is greater today than ever before. As shown by the 1998 outbreak, which encompassed twenty-two states, and the more recent 2002 outbreak, which encompassed seven states, a food produced in one location can reach many places across the country. When outbreaks are spread out across a broad area, they are harder to detect and harder to trace.

Also, today most animals bred for consumption are raised on huge farms and are processed in huge slaughterhouses, which critics say increases the chances for

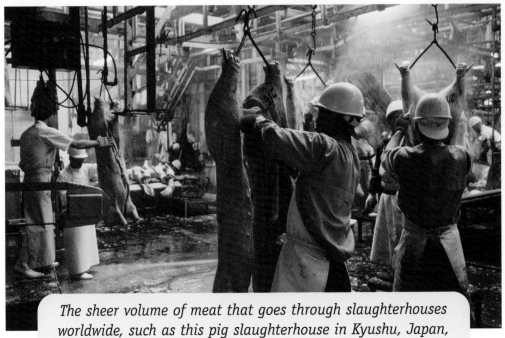

The sheer volume of meat that goes through slaughterhouses worldwide, such as this pig slaughterhouse in Kyushu, Japan, makes it very hard to contain threats like Listeria.

contamination. "The meat industry has gotten so huge and is processing meat at such a large volume in these huge slaughterhouses, it's easy for meat to become contaminated," said Navis Bermudez of the Sierra Club in an October 15, 2002, interview in the *New York Times*. "When these animals arrive at the slaughterhouses, their hides are already filthy with manure from being raised in such confined spaces," Ms. Bermudez said, "and they are likely to be stressed, which helps create more pathogens."

Finally, the number of people who would be vulnerable to listeriosis is growing as well. An increasing number of elderly people, coupled with an increasing number of people with chronic illness who can now be kept alive by advances in modern medicine, means that there will be more people who will be at risk of suffering the most serious effects of listeriosis.

As the government and scientists search for better ways to control this deadly bug, it is important that people in vulnerable groups be aware of what they need to do to avoid being exposed to this deadly illness. Educating the public about how they can protect themselves from listeriosis is an important focus of the government's plan to guard against this deadly disease.

LISTERIOSIS IN THE HOME

The CDC tells people at risk for listeriosis to exercise the following precautions against the disease when preparing food.

- Reheat until steaming hot the following types of ready-to-eat foods: hot dogs, fermented and dry sausage, and other deli-style meat and poultry products. Thoroughly reheating food can help kill any bacteria that might be present. If you cannot reheat these foods, do not eat them.

(Continued on page 54)

- Wash hands with hot, soapy water after handling these types of ready-to-eat foods. (Wash for at least twenty seconds.) Also, wash cutting boards, dishes, and utensils. Thorough washing helps eliminate any bacteria that might get on your hands or other surfaces from food before it is reheated.

- Do not eat soft cheeses such as feta, Brie, Camembert, blue-veined cheeses, or Mexican-style cheese. You can eat hard cheeses, processed cheeses, cream cheese, cottage cheese, and yogurt.

- Do not drink raw, unpasteurized milk or eat foods made from it, such as unpasteurized cheese.

- Observe all expiration dates for perishable items that are precooked or ready to eat.

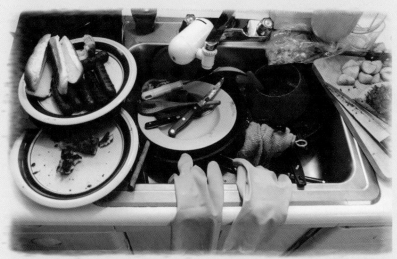

Exposing food to items that have touched raw meat and other raw products is a surefire way to risk contracting listeriosis and other food-borne pathogens.

GLOSSARY

assumption   The act of assuming or taking upon oneself.

contamination   Soiling or pollution by inferior material, as by the introduction of organisms into a wound or sewage into a stream.

DNA (deoxyribonucleic acid)   The molecule that encodes genetic information in the nucleus of cells. It determines the structure, function, and behavior of the cell.

epidemiologist   A person who is responsible for developing and monitoring activities for the surveillance, identification, and control of communicable diseases; a person who investigates epidemics or communicable disease outbreaks to determine the cause and probable sources.

epidemiology   The study of epidemic diseases.

Federal Drug Administration (FDA)   The U.S. Agency responsible for regulating biotechnology and food products.

meningitis   Infection of the meninges, which is the membrane that covers the brain and spinal cord.

microbe   A microscopic living organism, such as bacteria, protozoa, fungi, or virus, that is capable of causing disease in humans and animals.

microorganism   Any microscopic form of life, particularly applied to bacteria and similar organisms, especially those that are supposed to cause infectious diseases.

microscopic   Of extremely small size, visible only by the aid of a microscope.

miscarriage   The death of a fetus inside the mother's womb.

pasteurization   The heating of milk, wines, fruit juices, and so on, for about thirty minutes at 154°F (68°C) whereby living bacteria are destroyed but the flavor or bouquet of the liquid is preserved.

pathogen   Any virus, microorganism, or other substance that causes disease; an infecting agent.

psychrophilic   Able to grow at low temperatures as low as 32°F.

radiation   The process of emitting radiant energy in the form of waves or particles.

septicemia   Bacteria in the bloodstream, or blood poisoning; a disease affecting the body as a whole that is associated with the presence of pathogenic microorganisms or their toxins in the blood.

stillbirth   The birth of a dead fetus.

FOR MORE INFORMATION

Centers for Disease Control and Prevention
Public Inquiries/MASO
Mailstop F07
1600 Clifton Road
Atlanta, GA 30333
(800) 311-3435
Web site: http://www.cdc.gov

Food Safety and Inspection Service
U.S. Department of Agriculture
Washington, DC 20250-3700
(202) 720-8594
Web site: http://www.fsis.usda.gov

U.S. Food and Drug Administration
5600 Fishers Lane
Rockville, MD 20857-0001
(888) INFO-FDA (463-6332)
Web site: http://www.fda.gov

In Canada

Canadian Food Inspection Agency (CFIA)
59 Camelot Drive
Ottawa, ON K1A 0Y9
(800) 442-2342
Web site: http://www.inspection.gc.ca

Web Sites

Due to the changing nature of Internet links, the
Rosen Publishing Group, Inc., has developed an
online list of Web sites related to the subject of this
book. This site is updated regularly. Please use this
link to access the list:

http://www.rosenlinks.com/epid/list

FOR FURTHER READING

Caballero, Benjamin, and Barry M. Popkin. *The Nutrition Transition: Diet and Disease in the Developing World*. New York: Academic Press, 2002.

Fuller, Kristi. *Eating for Life: Boost Immunity, Prevent Disease, Celebrate Good Food*. New York: Books: 2001.

Marth, Elmer H., and Elliot T. Ryser, *Listeria, Listeriosis, & Food Safety*. New York: Marcel Dekker, 1999.

Ransley, J.K., J. Donelly, and N.W. Read. *Food and Nutritional Supplements: Their Role in Health and Disease*. New York: Springer Verlag, 2001.

INDEX

CREDITS

About the Author

Maxine Rosaler is a writer who lives in New York City.

Photo Credits